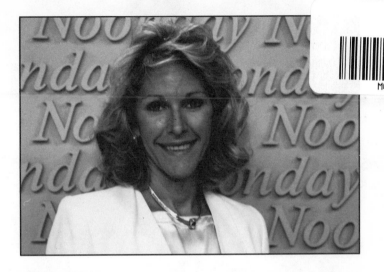

Dee Massengale lives in Atlanta, where she works with patients in orthopedic rehabilitation and physical therapy and maintains a private practice as a fitness trainer. She is a regular guest on 11-Alive *Noonday* presented by WXIA-TV, Atlanta's NBC affiliate, and is a professional consultant in back care for the Atlanta Sporting Club.

Dee holds masters degrees in exercise physiology and counseling psychology from Georgia State University. For the past four years, she has appeared on television newscasts, reporting on health and fitness issues. She also has produced a videotape, "The Exercise Alternative," in which she demonstrates biomechanically sound exercises that are especially useful for people with non-discogenic back problems.

THE GUIDE TO A
BETTER
BACK

A BACK PAIN SUFFERER'S HANDBOOK FOR EXERCISE AND DAILY LIVING

BY
DEE MASSENGALE, M.Ed.

SUSAN HUNTER
ATLANTA, GEORGIA

Published by Susan Hunter Publishing, Inc., Atlanta, Georgia.
Manufactured in the United States of America.

5 4 3 2

Publisher: Susan Hunter
Editor: Phyllis Mueller
Editorial Assistant: Nancy Kahnt
Design and Composition: 3x3 Studio
Line Art: Craig Luce

Library of Congress Cataloging-in-Publication Data

Massengale, Dee, 1956
The guide to a better back.

1. Backache — Exercise therapy. I. Title.
RD771.B217M37   1987   617'.56   87-31104
ISBN 0-932419-12-7

TO MY MOTHER, who stood by me emotionally, and took care of me physically during my year of incapacitation and rehabilitation.

CONTENTS

MY STORY

Running was my compulsion. For 7 years I put in 4 to 6 miles a day — every day — rain or snow. Then the pain began; excruciating lower back spasms that felt as if my lower spine was being ripped from my body. My years of improper weight lifting, aerobic dance, bending, twisting, and running on soft sand had caught up with me.

I spent my 26th birthday hospitalized and in traction. I was given demerol for pain and told that I would be all right in a week. I wasn't.

I remained at home in bed for the next three months unable to care for myself or drive a car. During this time I tried a virtual supermarket of remedies. There was biofeedback to see if the spasms were "in my head," numerous visits to two chiropractors, expensive accupuncture treatments, naturopathic salts and megadoses of vitamins, applications of DMSO, massage, and daily dips in a whirlpool.

Eventually, a wonderful physical therapist discovered I had sacro-iliac instability — joints that weren't holding together properly. Therapy involved pulling and pushing my joints back into line and strengthening the surrounding and supporting muscle groups.

It took 9 months. During this painstaking year, I was unable to sit for longer than 10 minutes before a wrenching muscle spasm would knock me back on to the floor.

I spent my time reading every book and article I could find on back pain and finished my master's degree in exercise physiology. I felt a strong need to turn what had been a painful and frustrating experience into a positive one. I wanted to share what I learned the hard way so others could prevent or nip in the bud what I went through.

If You Think You Can't, Read On!

Anyone who has ever had back pain fears it will return. A sedentary lifestyle may seem to be the safest way to avoid conflict with your body; after all, your doctor told you bedrest for 2 weeks. Any sign of strain or spasm sends you back to lying on the floor to "rest." Perhaps what no one ever told you was that tight, stiff, and/or weak muscles precipitate most spinal pain.

When I was first injured, I was a compulsive athlete. The more I was told to rest, the more I was determined to exercise. (No one should exercise during an acute attack of back pain.)

RX for Back Pain: Exercise

Regardless of the etiology or pathology, expedient rehabilitation and indisputable prevention are to limber the muscles that are tight, to strengthen the ones that are weak, and to follow proper body mechanics during your daily activities every day for the rest of your life. Exercise is arbitrary work, back pain is not.

This book is organized topically, and is divided into 8 parts. It's not necessary that you read the parts in any particular order, but it is important that you read parts 1-7 and consult with your physician before embarking on your exercise program.

Also, some language in this book is fairly technical and these definitions may be helpful:

body mechanics — the methods one uses and the positions one assumes in doing any physical task

etiology — the underlying cause of disease

herniation — the external protrusion of the innermost part of a disc

lordosis — the natural curve in the lower (lumbar) spine

microtrauma — small, injury-causing damage that can be progressive and lead to significant pathology

pathology — a diseased state, dysfunction

The purpose of this book and your goal are to find the exercises that work for you and do them religiously from this day forward. Back pain is analogous to addiction. You can be rehabilitated or reformed, but one slip and the disease and pain take over again. Keep this analogy in mind, and read, study, and live by the Cardinal Rules — Part 1.

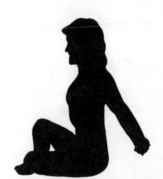

THE CARDINAL RULES

Get Plenty of Rest
Don't Arch Your Back
No Forward Bending
Keep Your Knees Bent
Never Twist and Never Bend and Twist
If It Hurts Don't Do It
Always Lift With Your Legs
Attain Your Ideal Weight
Avoid Activities That Compress the Joints

GET PLENTY OF REST

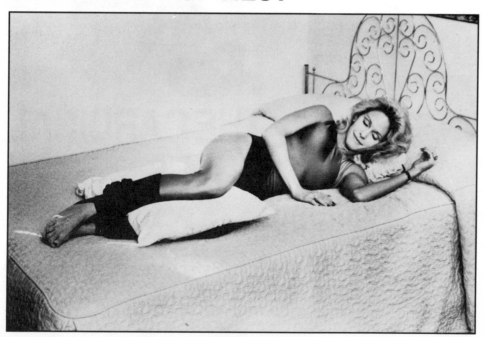

A joint is most vulnerable when the muscles that support it are tired. As the muscles fatigue, your body weight, the stress of movement, and gravity take their toll. Ligaments become overworked and stretched. You may have microtrauma, or even injury. If you feel too tired to exercise because you only got 5 hours sleep because the dog barked all night, do yourself a favor. Don't exercise; take a nap instead.

There is a proper way to rest. Most specialists agree that sleeping in the fetal position with a pillow between the knees is the best posture for slumber.

A firm mattress is also a must. Consider buying an orthopedic mattress, or insert a piece of plywood underneath your mattress to provide an unyielding surface. **Everyone should avoid sleeping on the stomach,** for this causes undesirable arching and compression in the lumbar spine.

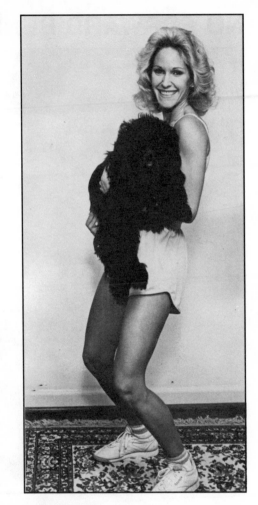

DON'T ARCH YOUR BACK

This applies to exercise and daily activities. Every time you arch your back you are compressing your lumbar discs, a perfect example of microtrauma. As the vertebra come together to compress the disc, a little fluid is lost each time. The disc begins to shrink. When you bend your knees and pull your pelvis forward, arching is prevented.

NOTE: When you have a heavy load in your arms the tendency is to lean back, but if you bend your knees this won't happen.

Remember: Always keep a pelvic tilt to avoid an increase in lordosis.

NO FORWARD BENDING

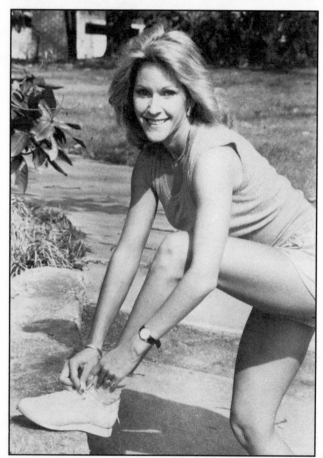

When you bend at an angle past 45°, you are literally hanging on your ligaments. Ligaments were not meant to stretch. (See the anatomy section, Part 2.) When you bend over to touch the floor, you are again sustaining microtrauma. Not only is this damaging to your ligaments, you are compressing lumbar discs. For example, if you have to tie your shoe, don't bend over from a standing position to reach your foot. Prop your foot in a chair. If you have to move down to the floor, use your legs: bend your knees and squat.

NOTE: When you have to cough or sneeze, stand up, bend backwards, bend knees, and increase lordosis to lessen the strain.

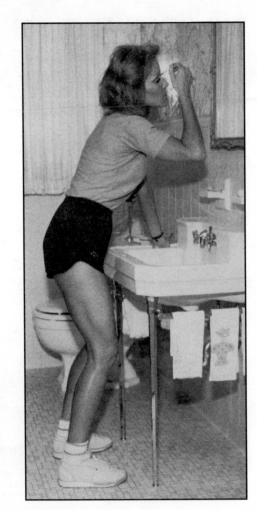

KEEP YOUR KNEES BENT

When you bend your knees (whether you are standing, lying on your back, or lying on your side) you are rotating the pelvis forward, maintaining normal lordosis (curve) in the lower back. This is important because the reverse posture, a swayback, puts enormous compression on lumbar discs and stretches and strains the spinal ligaments.

Example: Keep legs bent when standing at the sink to brush your teeth, wash your face, or apply make-up.

Remember: Keep knees bent when standing, lying flat, or lying on your side.

NEVER TWIST
AND NEVER BEND AND TWIST

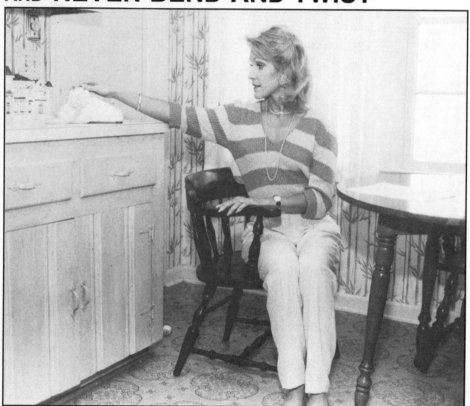

Twisting puts shearing stress on the lumbar discs. When your torso rotates but your hips are stationary, the vertebrae are rotating back and forth over the stationary discs. This is analogous to ringing out water from a wet towel. Many a disc has been ruptured while someone was leaning over and twisting the body or when coming up.

Example: When reaching for an object behind you while sitting in a chair, you always should rotate your hips to follow your shoulders to avoid twisting and rotational stress on the lumbar discs.

Remember: Turn your body, not just your head. Do not do complete 180-degree neck rotations. This movement places shearing stress on cervical discs. To loosen your neck, rotate your head to left and right and back again.

Pain is your body's signal that something is in trouble. You may be lying on your sofa when your back begins to hurt. Could it be the sofa is too soft and not providing adequate support? Get up and try lying on the floor.

If you are sitting in a chair (even one with excellent support) and your back begins to hurt, it is time to get up and walk around. I recommend that everyone get up **at least** once an hour. Sustained positions such as sitting tend to elongate the ligaments in the spine. These ligaments contain many nerve endings. When the nerve endings become irritated, pain results. Sitting applies enormous pressure on lumbar discs.

Standing for a lengthy period of time also can create strain in the lower back because, as a sustained position, it also is causing the ligaments to elongate. Keeping one foot raised a few inches will help relieve pressure. For example, if you are ironing or cooking, rest one foot on a low stool.

When possible, lie on the floor with your legs at a 90° angle over a chair. This position puts fewer pounds of pressure on your lower back than anything you can do.

IF IT HURTS, DON'T DO IT

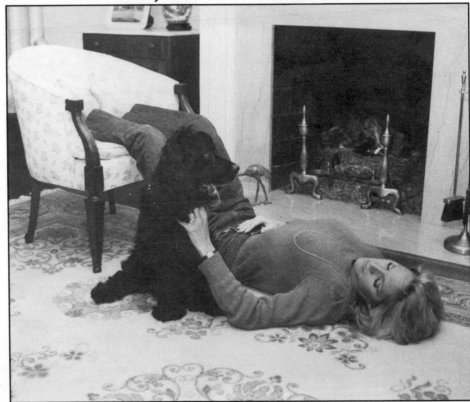

9

ALWAYS LIFT WITH YOUR LEGS

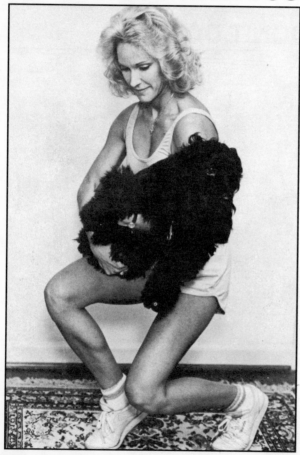

Regardless of the weight of what you are lifting, you must squat down. If the object is heavy, prop it on your thighs, then pull it toward your chest, and lift with a straight back. This will prevent forward bending and arching.

ATTAIN YOUR IDEAL WEIGHT

Extra body weight puts enormous compression on all joints, particularly the spine. More importantly, a protruding abdomen pulls on the spine, increasing the lordosis.

Abdominal exercises will strengthen, not spot reduce, a big belly. To reduce, you need to diet and exercise. Aerobic activities increase your metabolic rate and burn the most calories. My suggestions are stationary cycling, treadmill walking, brisk walking outdoors, and swimming. Everybody's fitness level is different. Ask your doctor or physical therapist how much time and what heart rate intensity is safe for you. (See Part 5 on aerobic training.)

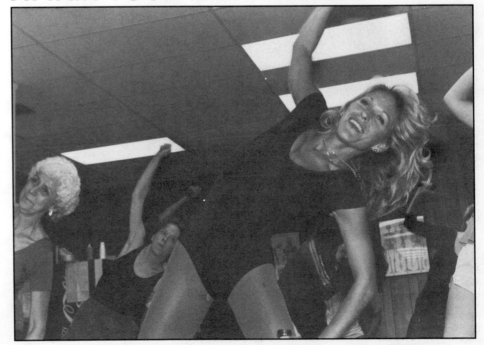

AVOID ACTIVITIES THAT COMPRESS THE JOINTS

These activities should be avoided by any one who suffers chronic or recurring back pain:

- Horseback riding
- Stationary running or jumping, such as aerobic dance
- Improper or heavy weight lifting
- Jumping rope
- Jogging
- Racquetball, handball, squash
- Tennis
- Basketball

Don't be discouraged. Look at what you can do!

- Swimming
- Brisk walking
- Power walking with hand weights
- Stationary bicycling
- The exercises in this book

The "can" list may be shorter, but take it from one who thought she would never walk again — they sure beat the alternative.

In order for you to better understand the remainder of this guide, it's important to understand the various aspects of the spine because they are the anatomical structures that we most often abuse from improper exercising or from faulty body mechanics. Their significance will be clearer after reading Parts 4 and 8.

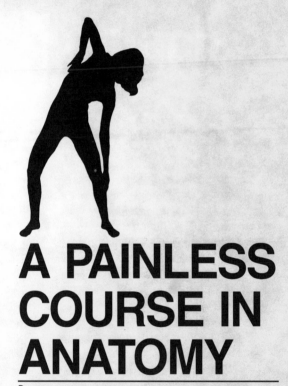

PART TWO

A PAINLESS COURSE IN ANATOMY

Bones
Joints
Discs
Ligaments
Muscles

FUNCTIONS OF THE SPINE

BONES (Osteology)

Lumbar Vertebrae. These are 5 separate kidney-shaped bones that form the lumbar curve in the lower back. With x-rays, a physician looks for pathology in and around the bone. Fractures, tumors, and osteoarthritis are detectable. However, soft tissue pathology (such as disc herniation, sprains, and strains) is not. You may have severe back pain and a perfect x-ray at the same time.

Cervical Vertebrae. These 7 bones form the neck. This also is a vulnerable area of the spine because of its ability to move in flexion, extension, rotation, and lateral bending.

Thoracic Vertebrae. These 12 bones make up the midsection of the spine. Because of the small curve in this region, almost all pathology is muscular in nature.

JOINTS (The Facets)

A facet is an articulation where 2 adjacent vertebrae meet to form a joint. The facet joints glide and are separated by synovial fluid, tissue, and cartilage. The direction (or plane) of the facet in any segment of the spine will determine the direction of movement permitted to that specific segment.

In a healthy back, each set of facets matches its neighbors in the next vertebra. A facet joint may become impinged or frozen, causing the muscles around it to spasm. It may even rest against a nerve, causing severe pain and restricting normal range of motion.

DISCS

A disc functions minimally as a shock absorber. Between each of the 33 vertebrae lies a sponge-like cushion that permits the spine to move into flexion (bending forward), extension (leaning back), and laterally (side to side bending). This fibrocartilagenous structure is composed of separate parts, an outer layer called the **annulus** and a central core called the **nucleus pulposus.** The disc contains 88% water and is held in a solution called the **matrix.**

Throughout the matrix are numerous layers of fiber that encircle the whole annulus to reinforce the disc. The many layers of annular fibers keep the vertebrae together and completely surround the central core.

14

The annular fibers can stretch to a limited degree. When the vertebrae are compressed together the fibers stretch, but do not tear. When the fibers are twisted (imagine unscrewing the lid of a jar), the fibers become stretched more than they can allow and tear. The outer fibers tear first and more completely than those in the layers closer to the center.

LIGAMENTS (To Restrict Motion)

A ligament is a taut, non-elastic, fibrous connective tissue that holds bone to bone. Ligaments are the stabilizers of a joint. Unlike muscles, ligaments don't return to their original length if and when they are severely stretched. Once a ligament elongates, the joint loses some of its stability. The bone or bones may

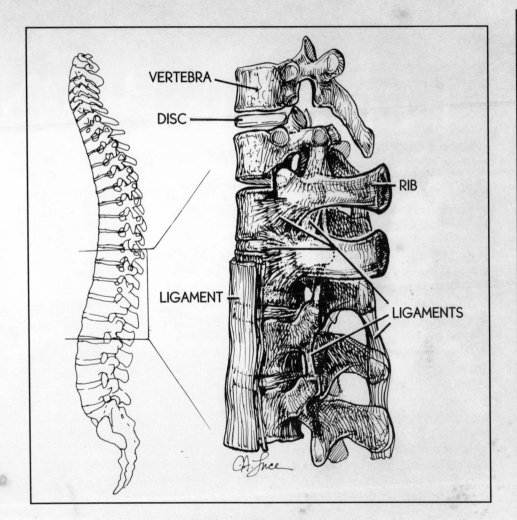

VERTEBRA

DISC

RIB

LIGAMENT

LIGAMENTS

move slightly, causing surrounding muscles to tighten or even spasm. There are numerous ligaments in the spine. The two longest, running from the cervical through the lumbar spine, are referred to as the anterior longitudinal and the posterior longitudinal. These ligaments play key roles in supporting the discs and preventing herniation. The lumbar spine has very narrow ligaments, so it is the most vulnerable area.

MUSCLES (To Initiate Motion)

A muscle is an elastic soft tissue with the capability of contracting and relaxing. There are over 400 muscles in the body. For a muscle to be toned or strengthened, it must be forced to contract or shorten. The reverse is true for a muscle to relax, it must be stretched or returned to its normal length. Muscles are susceptible to strains, tears, and "pulls" if they are not stretched properly or if they are overused.

In the back, there are 4 layers of very slow-contracting muscles. Due to their slow response time there is a high risk of strain to weak or tight muscles.

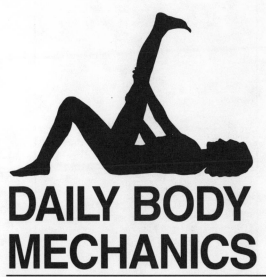

PART THREE

DAILY BODY MECHANICS

Posture
Sitting
Reaching
Making a Bed
Driving a Car
Removing Groceries from the Car
Gardening

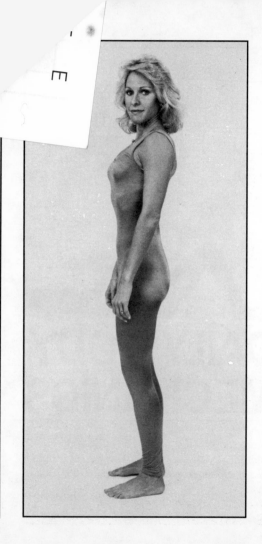

POSTURE

Sit proud and stand tall. Exercise is the only good way to improve strength and posture, and is our greatest weapon in the struggle against gravity. As the years pass, we have a tendency to lean forward; our muscles weaken and bone density decreases.

One very striking change is the humped back appearance in the thoracic spine, a condition aggravated by the loss of calcium from the bones. One reason the spine loses calcium is loss of muscle strength. The muscles across the front of the chest shorten and the shoulders tend to roll forward. To compensate for these changes in posture, the chin juts forward, tilting neck. Many of these changes can be delayed or even prevented with proper exercise.

The best postural alignment calls for a pelvic tilt. This is attained by pulling the abdomen in and squeezing the buttocks, while keeping the knees flexed or slightly bent. Keep your shoulders back, head straight.

SITTING

When you sit, use a firm pillow to support your lower back and prop your feet on a stool or phone book to support your lower back. By elevating the knees above hip level, you maintain a normal lordosis and decrease compression in the lumbar areas. Special lumbar support pillows may be purchased from your orthopedist or physical therapist. (Insurance will cover this expense.) This pillow should go with you to the movies, coliseum, stadium, and even restaurants. Any time you know that you will have to sit for more than an hour or on a hard surface, use your pillow. Don't be embarrassed. I take mine everywhere and no one has ever looked twice . . . so what if they do!

Choose a firm, high chair. Avoid sitting on low, soft chairs or sofas.

When you're getting up from a sitting position, try to maintain your lordosis.

When in acute pain, sit as little as possible, and then only for short periods of time.

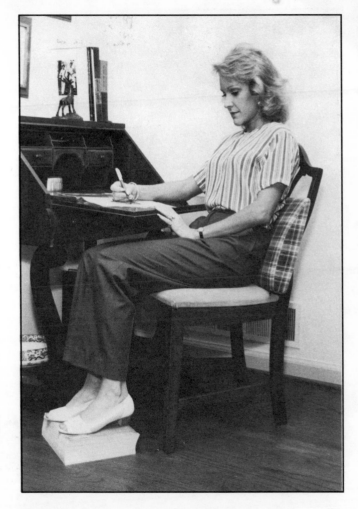

19

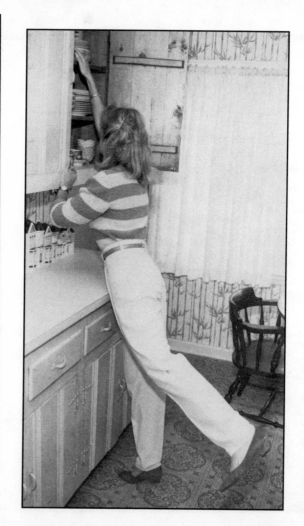

REACHING

Any time you reach straight up or overhead you arch your back, unless you extend one leg so that your back will remain flat.

MAKING A BED

You probably are accustomed to bending over to make your bed. Don't do that. Simply crawl on your knees to do the same job. Once you try it, you will find it is much easier. Best of all, you will not have any back pain while doing it.

21

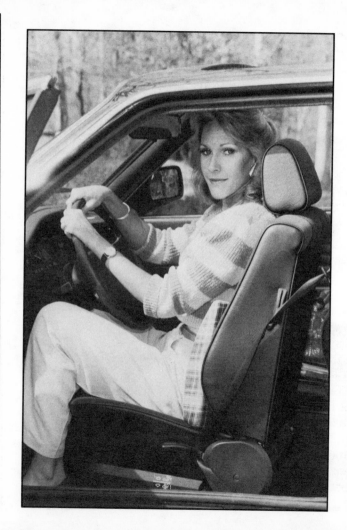

DRIVING A CAR

The best way to ensure proper posture while sitting is to keep the knees elevated above hip level to maintain the normal lordosis. In a car, this is done by pulling the car seat as close to the steering wheel as possible. Yes, your knees will feel like they are in your lap, but 30 minutes down the road you won't be feeling any (or as much) discomfort in your back! (Use your lumbar support pillow in the car, too, and **always** buckle your seatbelt.)

REMOVING GROCERIES FROM THE CAR

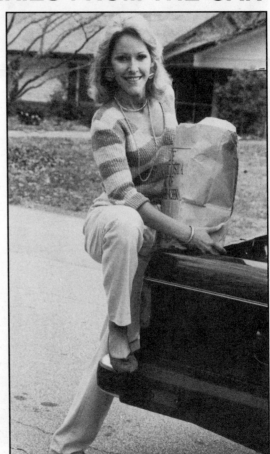

There are two body mechanics you must remember here, bend your knees and lift with your legs. Impossible? No! By propping one foot on the car bumper, you can reach for the bag without arching your back. Proceed by bringing the bag first to the edge of the car, slide it onto your thigh, and finally pull it toward your chest. You have not had to bend and lift. Tell the store clerk to put just a few items in each bag. It's better for your back to pick up four light bags than two heavier ones.

At the store, pull your heavy grocery cart, don't push it.

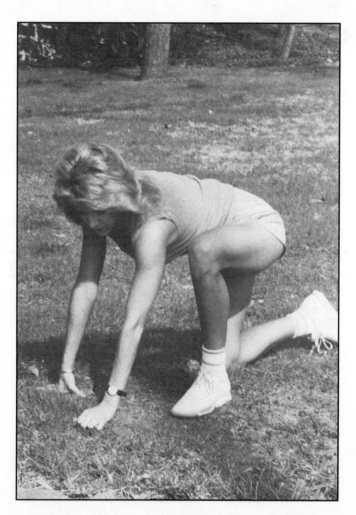

GARDENING

Gardening can be painful if proper body mechanics are not used. To avoid stooping, go down on all fours or rest on one knee with a flat back. In this position, your legs, and not your back, support the weight of your body.

Remember: Maintain a pelvic tilt with abdominal muscles contracted while pushing a lawnmower (or vacuum cleaner).

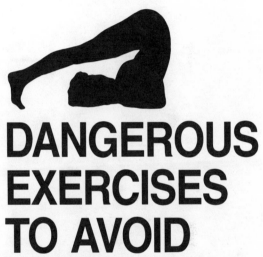

DANGEROUS EXERCISES TO AVOID

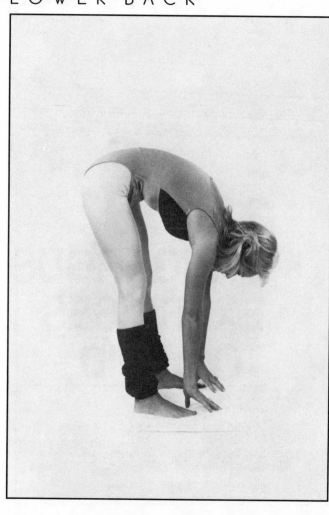

TOE TOUCH

This can put enormous strain on all of the structures in the lower back and stress back ligaments beyond normal limits. The muscles of the back cannot give you any support when you are toe touching, as you are actually stretching and hanging on your ligaments. Toe touching also puts a great deal of stress on the spine, as well as on the sciatic nerve, and can cause ruptured discs in an adult who has an underlying disc problem.

ALTERNATIVE

Lie on back with one knee bent and the other leg extended straight up (90° angle to the body); clasp hold of calf, pressing leg toward the body. Flex the foot and hold 20-30 seconds. This will stretch the back of the thigh. Do not bounce or force the leg forward.

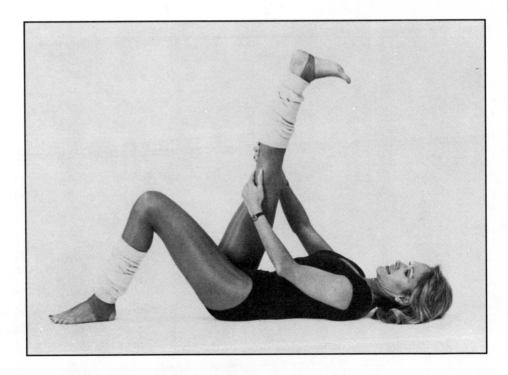

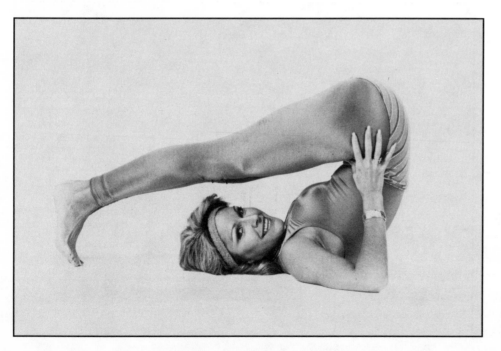

YOGA PLOW

The plow puts inordinate stress on blood vessels to the brain and upper spinal cord. In rare cases, strokes can occur due to the lack of blood circulation.

The plow is also bad for the back. It places a great load on the cervical vertebrae. At the end of the movement, when your feet are over your head, you are literally stretching the ligaments in your back.

This movement also approaches stretching the limits of nerve fiber length, creating the possibility of fiber injury to the sciatic nerve.

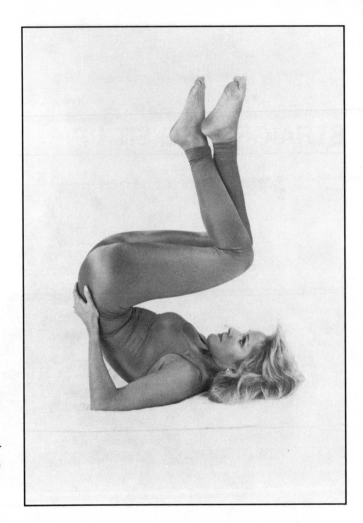

ALTERNATIVE
Place hands under the hips for support; point feet toward ceiling. Do not let body weight go past your shoulder blades!

STRAIGHT LEG SIT UP

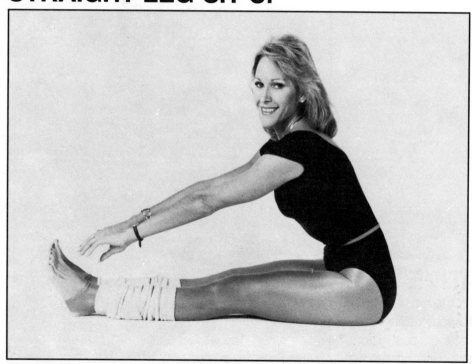

This exercise can result in back strain and abnormal elongation of nerves. The sitting position stretches the posterior longitudinal ligament beyond its normal anatomical bounds, and puts a great deal of stress on the sciatic nerve. The pelvis is rotated in an abnormal position, which exacerbates any sacro-iliac strain.

ALTERNATIVE

Bend knees, partially curl head and shoulders up. Do not rise up past the upright position, which can strain the back and elongate nerves. **Keep lower back on floor.** Keeping this small range of motion isolates the abdominal muscles, enhancing strength in the most efficient manner possible.

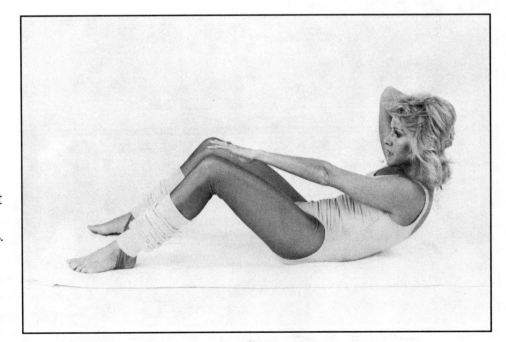

31

SIT UPS (with feet hooked)

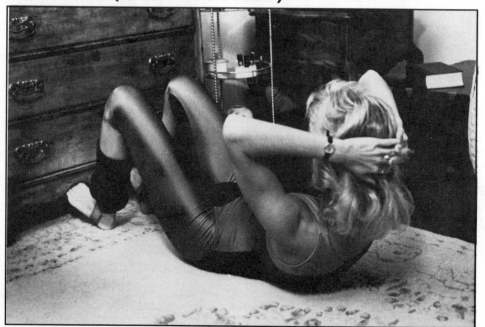

This sit up uses the hip flexor muscle in the upper thigh to pull up the body. When these muscles get tight, they pull the pelvis into torsion, compressing the fifth lumbar vertebra into the sacrum, increasing the lordosis and straining the muscles in the low back. This exercise is even more dangerous if done on an incline bench.

ALTERNATIVE (for the advanced exerciser)

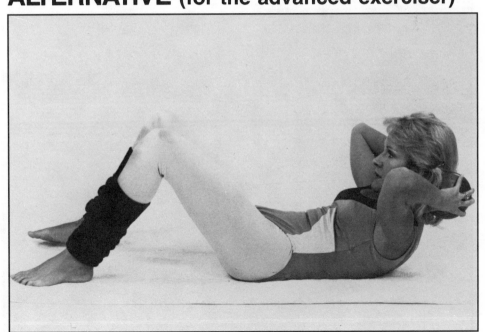

Mini-curl with a weight behind the head. Try to just lift the shoulder blades. The lower back must stay on the floor.

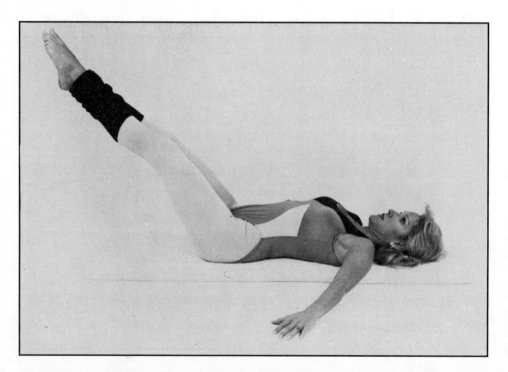

LEG RAISE

To lift both legs straight up and lower them without straining the back, you must **keep your spine completely on the floor.** During leg raises, the lower back is usually forced to arch. The weight of the extended legs then puts a tremendous amount of pressure on all the structures in your lower back.

ALTERNATIVE

Lie on back, place fists underneath buttocks, bring legs over head at right angles to the body, drop one leg at a time. Make sure one leg stays directly above torso. (This will keep the lower back from arching.) If it is too difficult to lower leg to the floor, try lowering it just half-way down. Bring leg straight up before alternating legs. **Exhale** as leg goes down.

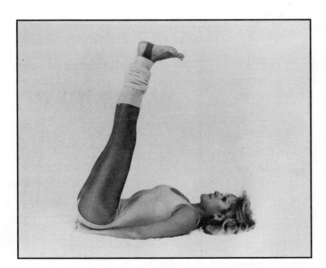

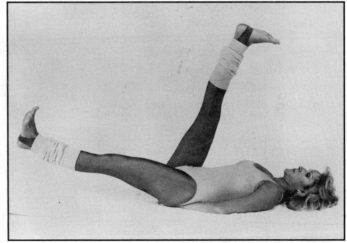

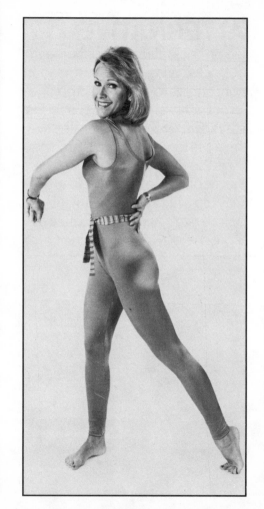

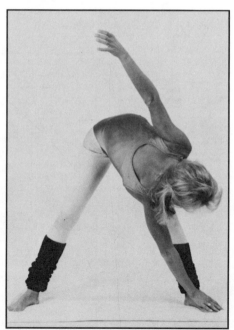

WAIST TWISTS

These movements put shearing stress on the discs of the lower back. Shearing, over a period of time, will decrease the discs' density, predisposing the lumbar region to degeneration and possible herniation. Twisting while bending is even more dangerous.

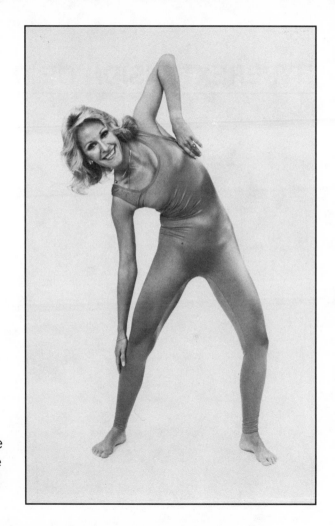

ALTERNATIVE

Do lateral side bends with **knees bent!** This is the only true way to work the oblique muscles of the waist. However, if you have acute disc disease, lateral bending should also be avoided.

HYPEREXTENSION OF THE BACK

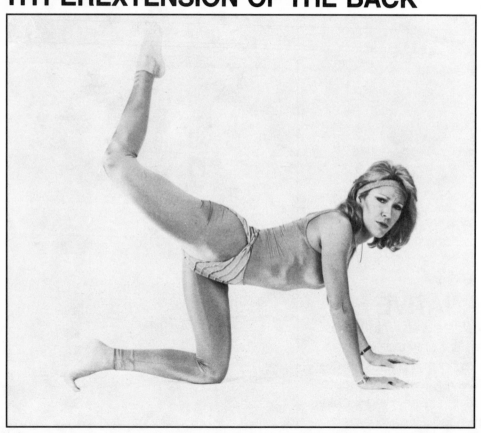

Again, discs are compressed and all soft tissues can be strained. Always avoid arching! Never lift leg higher than hip level on floor exercises, and always lift from elbows and knees, not hands and knees.

ALTERNATIVE

From elbows and knees, extend one leg straight back and flex the foot. Try not to bend your knee and lift leg from the floor to hip level very slowly. Do not let leg go higher than hip. (That will arch the back.) **Exhale** as you lift the leg.

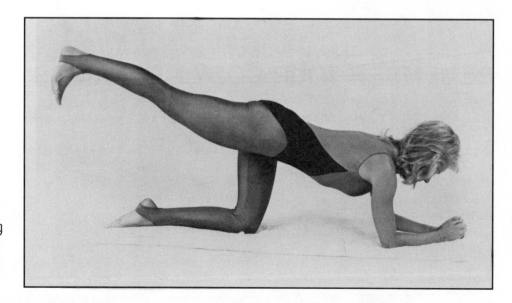

REMEMBER YOUR BODY MECHANICS

- Always keep knees bent when standing, regardless of the exercise. This will decrease your lordosis and take strain off the lower back.
- Maintain a forward pelvic tilt during all exercises. Remember to hold the abdomen in tight.
- Never jerk or do fast movements. Slow movements work the muscles more and are safer.
- A stretch is only a stretch if it is held for at least 20 seconds. Do not bounce or force the muscle, as it triggers a reflex that causes the muscle to tighten up.
- Always warm up for 5 minutes before any static stretching or vigorous activity. (See Part 5 for directions.)

A NOTE ABOUT WEIGHT LIFTING:

When lying on a bench to press or perform flies for the chest, pull your feet up on the bench or, even better, pull your knees to your chest; If you can't complete the lift or range with your knees up, the weight is too heavy for you, and you are compensating by using your back.

Always stretch your back before and after you lift weights.

If it hurts, don't do it.

Avoid doing any kinds of curls or sit ups on an incline board. The angle forces your hip flexors to do most of the work. The result? Enormous strain in the lumbar area.

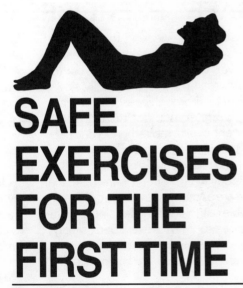

PART FIVE

SAFE EXERCISES FOR THE FIRST TIME

Flexibility
Strengthening
Aerobic Conditioning

"SAFE" EXERCISES FOR THE FIRST TIME

Biomechanically speaking, the following exercises are safe. This does not mean, however, that all of them will work for you. Approach each one carefully, slowly — only after thoroughly reading the directions. **Every** do and don't is extremely important. If any move hurts your back stop immediately, pull your knees to your chest and take a couple of deep breaths. Then cautiously proceed to the next one. There are as many as a hundred different possible pathologies in the spine and one exercise program for every body simply does not exist. Pain is your body's warning system. When it starts, you stop!

BEFORE YOU BEGIN, READ THIS

The first step to attaining flexibility is regaining normal range of motion in your joints. It is achieved through a static stretching routine.

Your second goal is to rebuild your strength which may have been lost through inactivity. The exercises will also tone your muscles and aid in recontouring your body. Many important stretching exercises are also in the second part of this chapter, "Strengthening." **Be sure to include these stretches in your flexibility routine.** You will be doing calisthenics, isometrics, and weight training.

Last, but certainly not least, you will embark upon an aerobic activity that will provide you with cardiovascular conditioning, endurance and energy. Aerobic activities help your body efficiently expend calories, which is important in weight management.

I have provided a small number of exercises for 3 reasons. First and foremost, there are only a few "safe" ways a back pain sufferer can perform calisthenics without risk of further injury. If one exercise works and is comfortable, then do 3 sets of that one instead of trying 2 additional exercises that may not be as comfortable. Second, the more you have to learn, the greater the chance that you won't pay attention to detail. Details are very important. Third, some exercises are not safe. Don't generalize.

FLEXIBILITY

Before you do any exercise, you should warm up; you literally raise the temperature of your muscles by increasing blood flow to them.

42

The increased blood flow enhances elasticity and flexibility of tendons, ligaments, and muscles and reduces the risk of pulls and tears. Blood saturation will also decrease lactic acid accumulation, decreasing the chances for muscle soreness later.

You can warm up actively or passively. An active warm up could be riding a stationary bike for 5 minutes, taking a walk, or "running" toe/heel in place for 3 minutes while you make circles with your arms. (By "toe/heel," I mean your feet never leave the floor.) If you are unable to do any active warm-up, you can achieve the same results by sitting in a whirlpool or a bathtub of hot water. **Remember:** Cold muscles don't stretch. Always take the time to warm up.

Flexibility is the ability to carry a joint through a **normal** range of motion without undue stress or damage. Many exercise books picture contortions and refer to them as stretches. You are not a yogi, and you probably aren't a gymnast, so please don't compare your abilities to theirs. A good rule of thumb is that if it looks unnatural, it probably is, so don't try it.

Flexibility is important in preventing injuries and degeneration of the joints. When we are under stress, experiencing pain, or performing any work task our muscles shorten. If they are not properly stretched, they become vulnerable to strains, tears, and painful spasms. An effective stretching program involves all the major muscle groups and joints of the body, not just the ones in your spine.

Tense muscles respond best to static stretching. This method is achieved by slowly moving into the stretch and holding it a minimum of 20 seconds. It is crucial that you don't bounce or force your stretch or the **stretch reflex** will result, and the muscle actually will contract and shorten instead of relaxing and elongating. Ballistic stretching is a forced movement that involves bouncing a muscle, and is definitely contraindicated. Bouncing can also cause muscle tears and trauma to the joint.

Flexibility tends to decrease with age. A well-rounded stretching program has been shown to counteract this decline and reduce the discomfort and incapacity associated with the aging process.

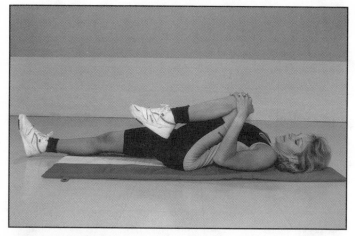

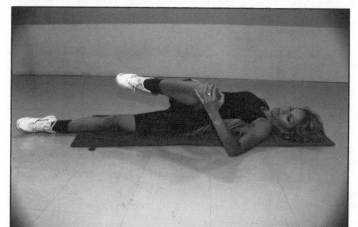

Do these exercises every morning and before and after any exercise routine. If doing these stretches causes you pain, **seek medical advice** before attempting **any** exercise. **NOTE:** Always proceed cautiously. Even though these stretches may be painless, the other exercises in this book may not be right for you. Your back is uniquely yours!

KNEE TO CHEST

Lie on your back, keeping one leg straight and pulling the other knee as close to your chest as possible. Hold 20 seconds and switch.

KNEE OVER

Lie on your back. Pull your knee to your chest, then gently pull your bent knee across your body, feeling the stretch in the muscles of your hip and back. Hold 20 seconds and switch.

KNEE OVER KNEE

Lie on your back. Cross your left knee over your right knee. Drop both legs to the left and raise your right arm above your head. Hold 20 seconds and switch.

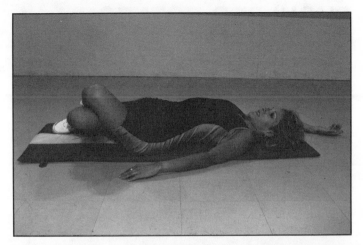

BOTH KNEES TO CHEST

Lie on your back. Pull both knees to chest, keeping your head and neck comfortably on the floor. Hold knees to the chest for 20 seconds. Release. Repeat 3 times.

Remember: You need to do all the stretches in the strengthening exercise section too! See the Leg Stretch (page 66), Hip Stretch (page 68), Hamstring Stretch (page 70), and Inner Thigh Stretch (page 72). These stretches also should be done after any aerobic activity, such as walking or biking.

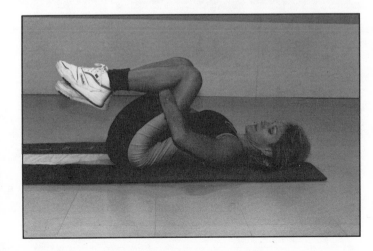

SHOULDER ROTATION

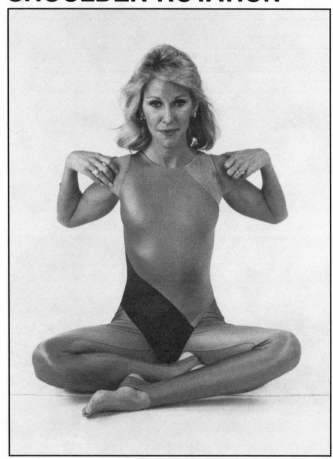

Hands on shoulders, draw a large circle with bent elbows. Try to lift the shoulder blades up, press back and down. Do 4 circles to the front, 4 to the back. This loosens the muscles in the shoulder and shoulder blade areas.

RANGE OF MOTION

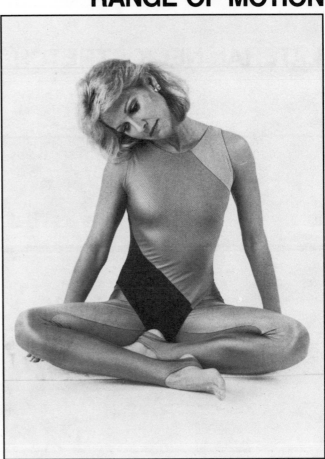

Drop the chin toward the chest. Rotate and side bend neck either left or right. At the end of range of motion, hold the stretch for 10-15 seconds. Repeat. This loosens the neck.

NOTE: Never rotate the head all the way back. This 360° range will place shearing stress on your cervical discs.

LATERAL NECK STRETCH

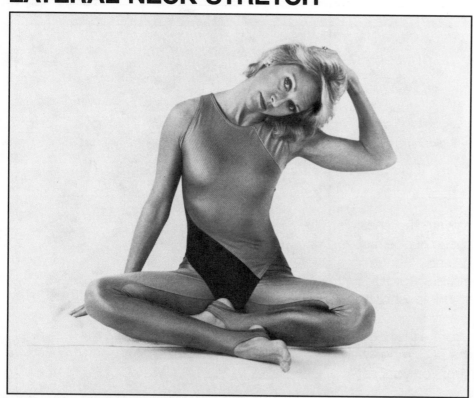

Drop shoulders down, sit up straight, gently pull head so that the left ear is pressed toward the left shoulder. Hold 6 seconds, repeat on right side. Repeat one more time. This stretches the muscles in the side of the neck.

DIAGONAL NECK STRETCH

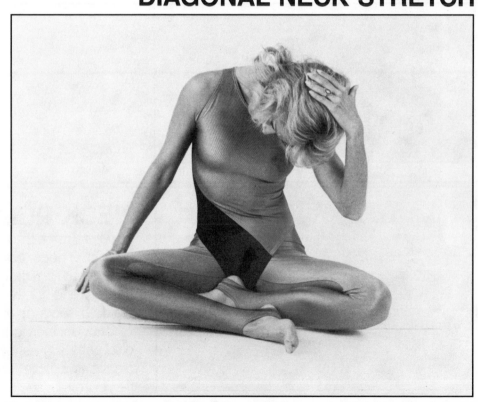

Drop shoulders, complete the lateral stretch (from the previous page). Then drop chin down toward chest and pull head forward. Hold 6 seconds and repeat on other side. This stretches the muscles that run in between the back and side of the neck.

49

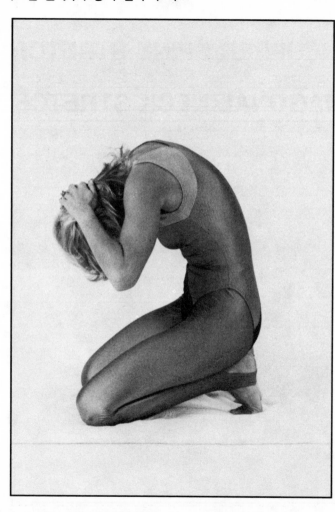

NECK PULL

Always stretch the neck and upper back after upper body strengthening exercises. Simply press the head forward and gently round the spine. Hold 15 seconds and repeat.

Caution: Individuals with known disc pathology should consult a physician before attempting this flexion exercise.

UPPER SPINE STRETCH

From knees, in a kneeling position, criss-cross hands and arms behind shoulders, **hold stomach muscles in tight,** lean forward, shift hips to right and lean upper torso to the left. Hold 6 seconds and shift to other side. This stretches the upper and lateral back.

Caution: Individuals with known disc pathology should consult a physician before attempting this or any other flexion exercise.

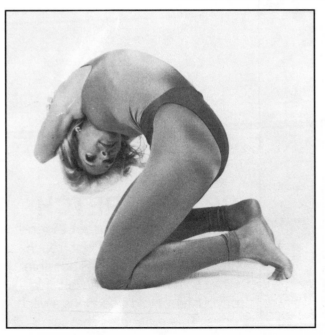

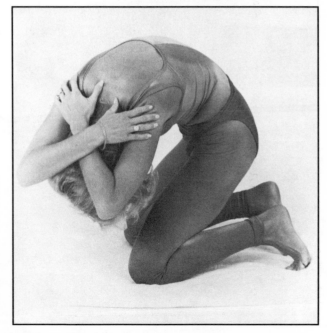

51

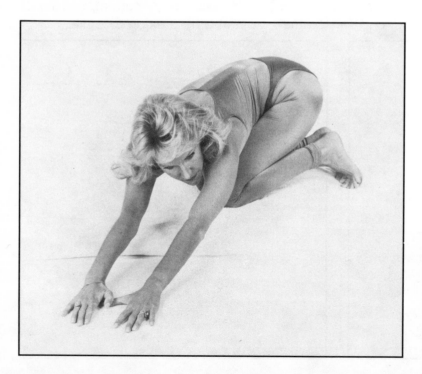

SPINE STRETCH

From feet, sit back on feet, extend arms straight out in front, reach arms as far to the right as possible while shifting seat to the left side of your feet. Hold 6 seconds, switch sides. This elongates the spine.

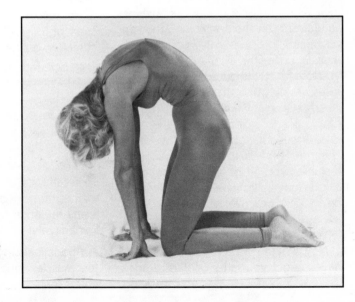

CAT ARCH

On hands and knees, let head and neck relax and pull stomach in toward spine. Simultaneously, lean body toward thighs to increase the stretch. Hold 6 seconds. Repeat 3 times.

53

STRENGTH

Let's first look at what happens to a muscle when it isn't exercised. We initially have muscles that are lean, with very little fat. As we become more sedentary, fat invades the muscle until it becomes so saturated it can't hold any more. Then the fat begins to accumulate outside the muscle, under the skin. When you diet, you lose fat on the outside of the muscle. It is not until you exercise that you burn intramuscular fat, the fat inside the muscle. Obviously, loss of fat outside the muscles, or subcutaneous fat, will result in change of body size. The body becomes a smaller version of itself; for example, a body may go from being a big pear to being a little pear. Definition and firmness are a result of strengthening exercises, which help burn intramuscular fat.

Now that the possible esthetic results have caught your attention, remember the most important reason you are doing strengthening exercises is for your back! Exercise is a means of developing control over your back pain and helping prevent acute attacks.

For maximum results perform 3 sets just short of muscle fatigue. (Be sure to stretch in between sets.)

Muscle fatigue is the point at which your muscles become so tired that you can no longer do the exercise **properly.** This means you must stop **BEFORE** you cramp, strain, force, or use momentum to complete the range of motion.

Exercise is **not** a means of treating an acute attack that has already occurred; for that, the remedy is rest. **Remember: If any exercise hurts your back, stop immediately!**

Abdominals. By far, the most important muscle group to keep strong are the abdominals. These are the muscles that actually support the spine. If they are weak, the back must work overtime to keep you erect.

There are 3 primary abdominal muscles. The **rectus abdominis** runs vertically from the pubic crest to the 5th rib. The **obliques** run diagonally from the iliac crest (hip) to the last 3 ribs. The **transverse abdominis** runs horizontally from the iliac crest (hip) through to the xiphoid process (tail end of the sternum or breast bone).

Due to the various directions and placement of these muscles, several abdominal exercises are required. Select one exercise per muscle group. Perform 3 sets using maximum effort, stopping short of muscle fatigue.

Before you begin your abdominal routine, learn the stretch on the next page!

When your abdominal muscles become tight and the lift is too difficult to perform, you should roll over and extend your arms straight out in front, lifting only your chest, prop on hands and elongate tight abdominal muscles. This will allow you to do another set.

NOTE: To avoid arching your back, keep belly on the floor.

THE ABDOMINAL STRETCH

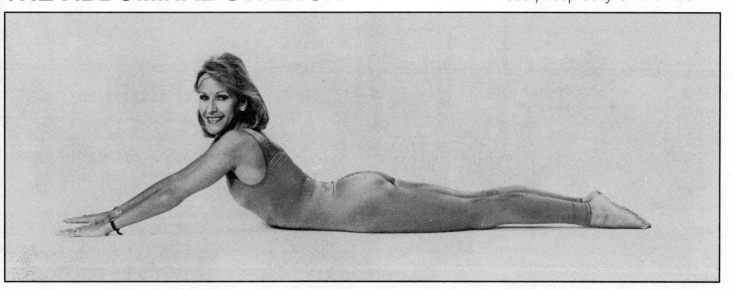

55

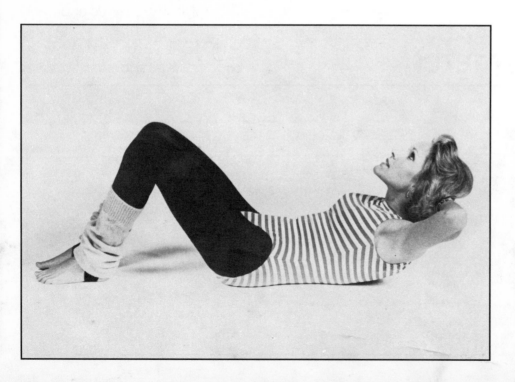

MINI CURL
Rectus abdominis
Lie on back, both knees bent, place hands **behind head** (never behind neck), keep elbows pressed back and parallel to the floor. Look directly toward the ceiling, chin up, and try to lift shoulders. **Exhale** as you lift.

   NOTE: You will not be able to lift very far.

SCISSORS

Rectus abdominis

Lie on back, hands behind head, elbows forward, legs straight up, scissor legs back and forth maintaining lower back firmly on floor. Do not let legs drop forward or back will arch. **Exhale** as the legs cross.

NOTE: This also works the transverse or lower abdominals.

Caution: If your hamstrings (muscles in the back of the leg) are so stiff that you cannot straighten them, omit this exercise.

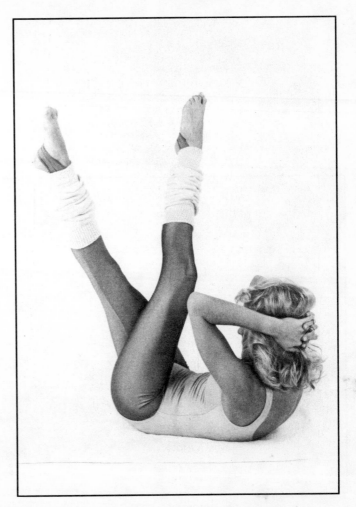

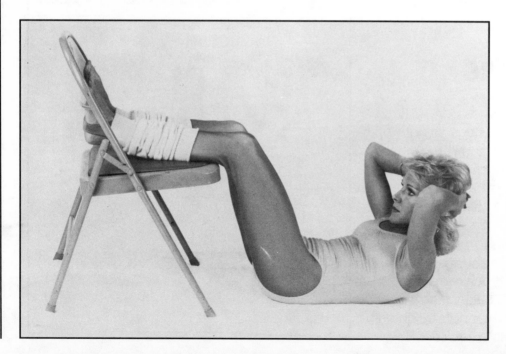

90°/90°
Rectus abdominis
Lie on back, place calves over a chair so that your legs form two right angles. With hands behind head, elbows forward, chin on chest, press forward. **Exhale** as you lift.

CURL WITH ONE ARM OUT IN FRONT

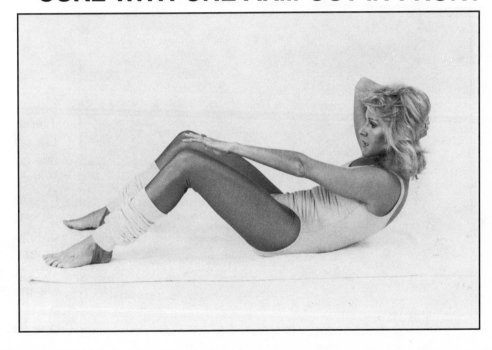

Rectus abdominis

Lie on back, both knees bent, one hand behind head, one hand straight out in front. To avoid neck strain, place chin on chest and leave it there. Lift shoulders off floor as your starting position, lift 3-4 inches. Wrist of extended arm should not extend past knees. Keep lower back on floor. This is a curl, not a "sit up". **Exhale as you lift.**

Caution: Omit if you have disc disease.

59

ELBOWS TO KNEES

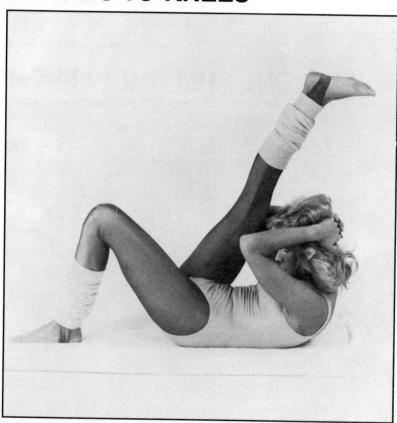

Transverse abdominis
Lie on back with one knee bent,
the other leg extended on floor.
With hands behind head, lift straight
leg up, and simultaneously bring
elbows forward lifting leg. **Exhale**
as leg comes forward. Repeat 10
times. Then use your other leg for
10 repetitions. Alternate until muscle fatigue. If this is too difficult,
place fist under seat and simply lift
one leg at a time.

SEAT LIFT
Transverse abdominis

Lie on back, grip floor covering or mat, keep head on floor, bend knees, lift seat approximately 4" off the floor. Try not to use momentum. The slower the movement, the more you will contract the lower abdominal muscles.
Exhale as knees come to chest.

   NOTE: If this movement is not possible, you may extend your arms over your head and clasp the legs of a chair. In this manner, your arm strength can be used to help you lift your seat.

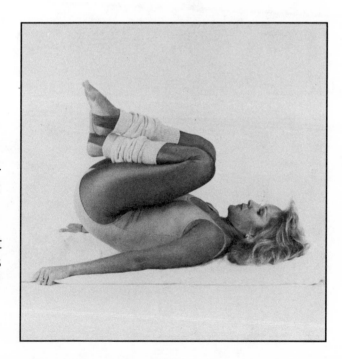

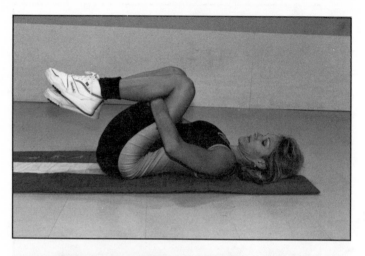

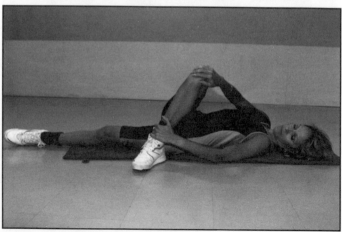

BACK STRETCHES

Stop now and stretch you back again. Lie on your back. Pull both knees to your chest, keeping your head and neck comfortably on the floor. Hold for 20 seconds and release. For the second stretch, extend your left leg. Pull your right knee to your chest. Then pull your right foot across your body, until you feel the stretch in your hip.

SIDE CRAWLS
Obliques

Standing with **both knees bent,** feet shoulder distance apart, reach right hand for right armpit. At the same time press right elbow directly toward the ceiling. Do not lean forward. Keep a pelvic tilt. Keep your right shoulder pressed back while reaching. **Exhale** as you reach. Repeat 10 on each side. Perform 2-3 sets.

   Caution: Consult with your physician or physical therapist before doing **any** lateral bending if you have disc disease.

   NOTE: If your back is weak, prop your extended hand on your knee to support your body weight.

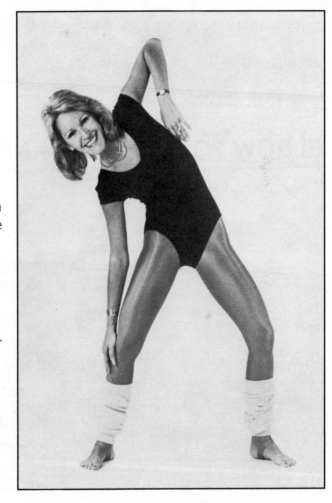

ELBOW TO OPPOSITE KNEE

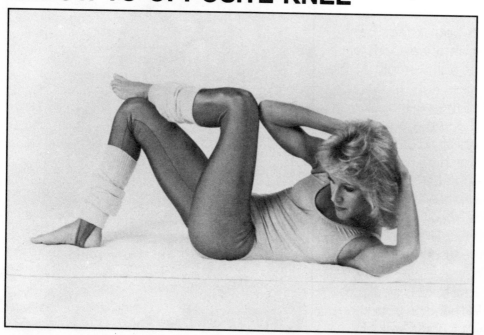

Obliques

Lie on back with knees bent. Place right foot on left knee. Hands behind head, bring left elbow to right knee. **Exhale** as you lift. Repeat 10 times, alternating legs until muscles are fatigued.

   NOTE: To make this more difficult, extend right leg straight up and then bring left elbow up and across.

Legs. Your legs must be strong so you can lift with them. If they cannot support your weight lifting from a squat, you will be forced to lean forward, calling on your spinal muscles to finish the lift.

WALL SIT

This is one exercise that is safe to do until it really hurts. There is no joint involvement so muscle fatigue is not dangerous. Place your back against a wall and slowly slide your feet out until they are just out past the knees. Drop your seat to a point just above hip level (**never** lower or you will compress the cartilage in your knees). Hold until muscles are fatigued, then slide up the wall, and stretch your legs (see next page for stretch).

Time yourself the first time to see how long you last.

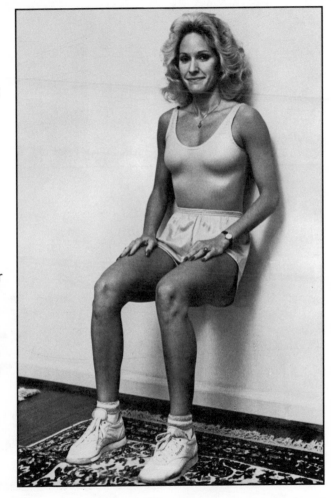

65

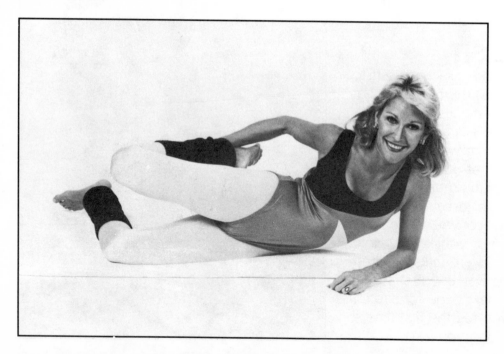

LEG STRETCH

Lie on your side, bottom leg bent, pelvis forward. Pull foot to your seat, but do not arch your back. Hold 20 seconds, repeat on the other leg.

SIDE LEG RAISES

Lie on your side, bottom leg bent, hips forward and stacked one atop the other. Extend top leg straight out, knee facing straight forward, flex the foot and lift 6″ from hip level. Repeat 3 sets stopping short of muscle fatigue. The lateral thigh muscles are important in pelvic stabilization. This is a particularly good exercise for those suffering from sacro-iliac instability. It also attacks "saddlebags" or bulging thighs.

IMPORTANT: Don't let leg drop below hip level. Strength and toning results will be more apparent. Be sure and stretch in between sets ! (See next page.)

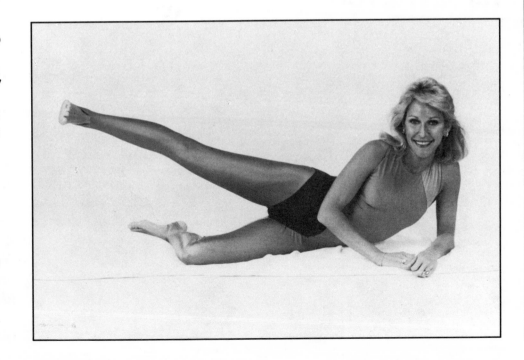

HIP STRETCH

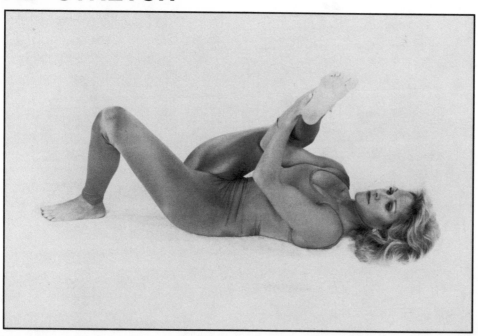

Lie on your back, bend right knee and pull calf toward chest. Make sure foot remains higher than knee to avoid compressing the cartilage in the knee joint. Hold 5-20 seconds, repeat on left leg.

NOTE: If you find this muscle to be extremely tender, try placing a tennis ball under the buttocks at the exact tender location of the muscle. Lean all of your weight on to the ball. This pressure will help inhibit muscle spasm and assist the muscle in relaxing. You should lie down to do this so that you can shift your weight according to the degree of discomfort you feel.

DONKEY LIFT

From elbows and knees **(never hands and knees),** extend one leg straight back. Flex foot. Try not to bend your knee and lift leg from the floor to hip level very slowly. Do not let leg go higher than hip. (This will arch the back.) **Exhale** as you lift the leg.

NOTE: Muscle Balance is important. The hamstrings or back of the leg must be worked to maintain a muscle balance with the strength of the front of your legs. If the muscles in the front of your legs are more than 60% stronger than your hamstrings, the alignment of your pelvis may be affected. As most back pain sufferers know, the hamstrings often become very tight. Your stretching is even more important while working these muscles. Don't let them cramp. If you are already very tight, perhaps it is best not to approach muscle fatigue. That is, do fewer repetitions than you otherwise would and increase the sets to 5. Stretch 20 seconds on each leg in between sets!

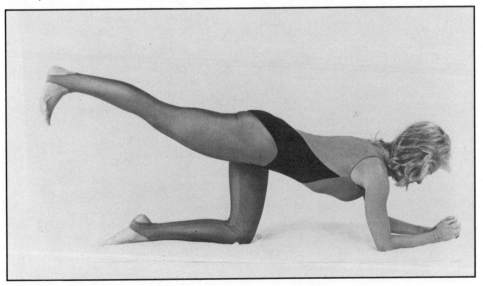

HAMSTRING STRETCH

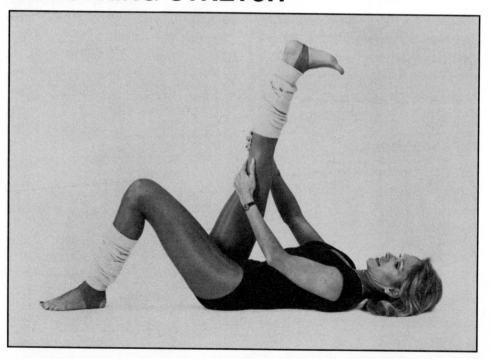

Roll over on back. With one knee bent, extend leg you need to stretch, wrap towel around your calf or grasp with hands and pull it forward until you feel the stretch. Do not bounce or force your leg. Hold at least 20 seconds.

Caution: If you have disc disease, you should stretch your hamstrings by propping your foot on a stool (2 feet is an appropriate height) and, keeping a flat back, gently lean forward until you feel the stretch in the back of your thigh.

KNEE SQUEEZE

This exercise works the inner thigh. Lie on back, grasping seat in hands. Bend knees and bring legs to a right angle to your torso. Open legs out, then pull knees back together. The key is to keep the knees and feet on the same plane, parallel with each other. Repeat 3 sets of 15. Stretch in between sets.

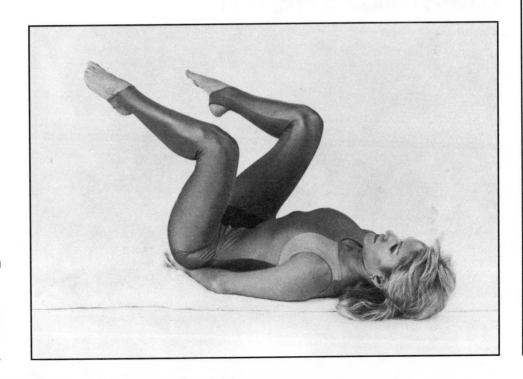

INNER THIGH STRETCH

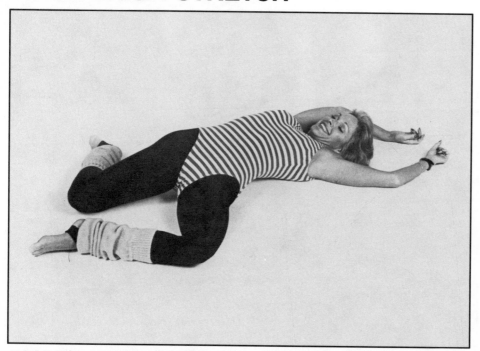

Lie on your back with knees bent. Place feet on the floor, shoulder distance apart. Drop knees to one side and hold for 20 seconds. Feel the stretch in your inner thigh. Repeat on other side. This also stretches your hip flexors and your back.

PELVIC TILT

This exercise works many muscle groups. When performed according to directions, you will contract the buttocks, quadriceps (muscles in the front of the thigh), calf, and pelvic floor muscles.

Lie on your back, knees bent and feet in front of knees. Come up on your toes and lift your seat. Make sure lower back stays on floor. Contract buttocks, and keep them tight, as you slowly tuck pelvis forward. The lift is very subtle and controlled. It is important that you don't arch your back. Try continuous tucks for one minute and work up to 3 minutes.

TO STRETCH: See Hip Stretch, page 68.

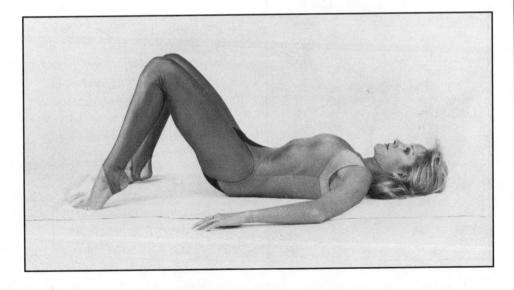

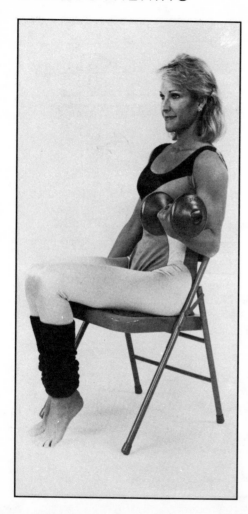

Upper Body. It is very important to have strength in your arms and chest to lift heavy objects, open heavy doors or do yardwork. Remember, if your primary mover muscle group isn't able to complete a task, your back will have to.

BICEP CURL

Sit in a chair, hold stomach in tight. Place a weight in each hand. Slowly raise forearms forward, extending the arms to complete the exercise. The weight needs to be heavy enough to fatigue your arm at 10-20 repetitions. Repeat 2 times, working up to 3 sets. This works the front of the arms.

NOTE: Experiment with various weights at a sporting goods store before purchasing. Women will probably start with 6 to 12 pounds and men 12 to 20 pounds. It is important that you do this exercise seated, so that you avoid arching your back. **Exhale** as arm comes forward.

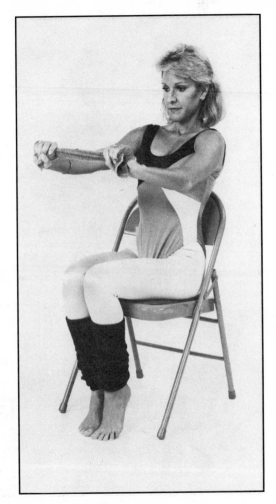

ARM EXTENSION

Sit in a chair and wrap a towel around your hands. With arms directly in front of chest, slowly bend elbows and bring hands toward body. Follow through by completely extending arms in front. Repeat 10 times, working up to 3 sets. Exhale as you extend arm. Keep the resistance as tight as possible. Arms should quiver. This exercise primarily works the pectoralis muscles in the chest.

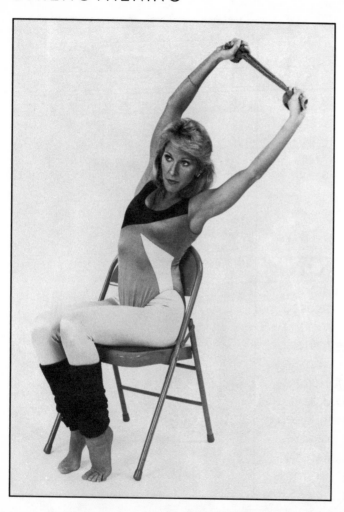

TRICEP EXTENSION

Sit in a chair, wrap a necktie, belt, or towel around your hands so that your arms are shoulder distance apart. Start with elbows bent; extend arms to one side. Keep arms behind ears, don't let arms drop forward, and don't arch. If you find yourself arching your back, try sitting on the edge of the chair. Hold stomach in tight! Your towel should not have any slack. Do 10 repetitions to each side. Work up to doing 3 sets. **Exhale** as you extend the arms. This exercise works the back of the arms.

NOTE: Working against your own resistance is an isometric function and can be as difficult and as beneficial as you make it.

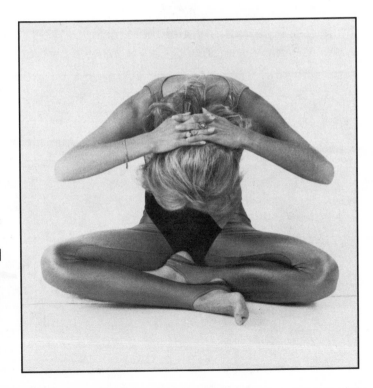

NECK PULL

Always stretch the neck and upper back after upper body strengthening exercises. Simply press the head forward and gently round the spine. Hold 15 seconds and repeat.

Caution: Individuals with known disc pathology should consult a physician before attempting this flexion exercise.

STRENGTHENING

Back. Are you wondering where the back exercises are? Actually the best thing you can do to strengthen your back is to walk, swim, or jog in a pool! If you choose to jog in a pool, stay in shoulder deep water with arms immersed. Try to push through the water as if you were running. Of course, you won't move very fast, but this is a great way to get your heart rate up and contract deep back muscles.

The following exercise will strengthen your back. Try it. If you have difficulty maintaining your balance, you need it. If you don't have a problem, omit it.

BIRD DOG

Begin on hands and knees, hold stomach in tight. Simultaneously lift right arm and left leg. Hold one second and switch. Keep head level with body. To increase difficulty, perform this exercise lying on your stomach with a pillow under your pelvis. Do 3 sets of 10, followed by the Spine Stretch (page 52).

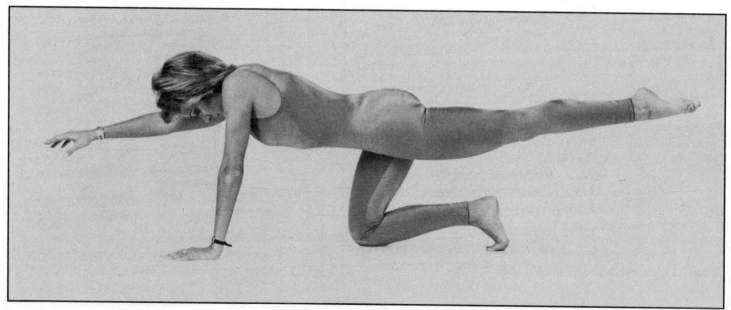

AEROBIC CONDITIONING

Aerobic exercise is steady, uninterrupted exercise that elevates your heart rate to its training zone for 20 minutes or longer.

Aerobic exercise is the most effective way to increase the metabolic rate and burn fat. The word aerobic means air or (more specifically) oxygen. Muscles need oxygen to perform. We can measure how hard a muscle is working by how much oxygen it uses. We can indirectly measure oxygen uptake by increases in heart rate of an exercising person.

Your "training zone," the minimum heart rate required to obtain cardiovascular benefits and the maximum safe heart rate to complete the activity, depends on your condition. For example, a 40-year-old individual who has not exercised in years and is 15 pounds overweight might have a training zone of 60-75% of maximum heart rate. His training heart rate is determined by using this formula:

Training Heart Rate Zone:

$$\begin{array}{r} 220 \\ -\ 40 \quad \text{(age)} \\ \hline 180 \ \text{maximum heart rate possible} \\ \times\ .60 \ \text{minimum heart rate to train} \\ \hline 108 \end{array}$$

$$\begin{array}{r} 180 \\ \times\ .75 \\ \hline 135 \ \text{maximum heart rate to train} \end{array}$$

As an individual gets into better physical condition, the training zone may increase to 75-85% of maximum heart rate ability.

If you haven't exercised strenuously in the last year and you are over 35, or have any personal history of heart disease or diabetes, you need to have a physical and perhaps a stress test before engaging in aerobic activity. Have your doctor or exercise physiologist suggest a safe training zone for you.

If you are under 35 and in good health you may begin at 70% and work up to 80-85% of your maximum heart rate.

Duration (length of time) is as important as intensity. For optimal results, I suggest the following. Of course, you may participate longer!

Brisk walking 30-45 minutes **or**
Brisk walking with 2-3 lb. hand weights, 20-30 minutes **or**
Non-stop swimming 20-30 minutes **or**
Stationary cycling 18-25 minutes.

NOTE: If you find it too uncomfortable to sit on your stationary bike for 20 minutes, you can combine cycling with walking. In other words, quickly leave your bike after

79

a 10 minute ride and immediately begin a 20 minute walk. Your heart rate will stay up and you will get your workout in without aggravating your back.

Progression is the key to progress. You may be able to do 5 minutes of your activity the first week. That is okay, as long as you add 2-3 minutes per week until you reach your goal.

Frequency is the last important fact for you to consider. To make significant progress and actually obtain cardiovascular benefits, you must do aerobic exercise at least 3 times per week. But why not make it a daily habit? Strive for 5-6 days per week! The results will be well worth the time and effort.

Aerobic exercise improves general fitness by providing a smoother flow of energy to the muscles. Physical activity feeds on adrenalin which, during periods of immobility, tends to accumulate in the heart and brain. The "grogginess" you may feel after what has seemed to be a hard day's work may be the result of a system that is like a car that has been "flooded" with gas, but not driven. Exercise, in a sense, burns your system clean of that residue, leaving you feeling refreshed. Inactive muscles build up strong electrified charges that can keep you awake. If you exercise, you can discharge these voltages and relax.

Aerobic exercise benefits the heart by helping it work more efficiently. With regular exercise, the heart pumps blood with less effort and it has more time to rest between beats. You can exercise longer without getting tired and respond to physical and emotional crises (stresses) without racing your heart or elevating blood pressure. Regular aerobic exercise can also reduce elevated blood pressure and elevated blood lipids (cholesterol), and the associated risks of "type A" personality. New blood vessels are produced which may provide enough circulation to replace that blocked by a plaque-choked artery.

By improving circulation, exercise improves brain functioning. It is our central nervous system, via the brain, which coordinates and regulates our glands, muscles, and other organs. The nervous system also directly or indirectly conditions behavior and consciousness.

We have an increased resistance to infection as a result of a stronger immune system. Increased circulation provides drainage of wastes and infection out of the body.

Blood sugar regulation is significant to both the diabetic and hypoglycemic individual. Aerobic exercise improves glucose tolerance. For the diabetic, this means that tissue sensitivity to insulin is increased. To the individual suffering from hypoglycemia or low blood sugar, change is seen in the oxidation of free fatty acids (for energy), so that glucose is stored rather than depleted.

Aerobic exercise can dramatically change your appearance. This primarily is due to an increase in the basal metabolic rate. BMR refers to the amount of energy (calories) required per hour to sustain life at rest with no physical activity. After aerobic exercise of at least 20 minutes duration, the BMR is raised for approximately 6 hours. This means that your body continues to burn calories at a faster rate than it would if you had not exercised. This increased caloric expenditure results in a change in body composition, if you don't increase your food intake. (Body composition is the ratio of adipose or fat tissue to lean mass — muscles and bones.)

All in all, you look and feel better, healthier, younger — all important in self esteem. The psychological and physical effects of improved fitness clearly go hand in hand.

POWER WALKING

Walking with 1 to 2 pound hand weights is a back pain sufferer's answer to jogging. The added weight and resistance of the weights increases the heart rate above that of regular walking. By keeping the elbows bent and pumping the arms you are also working the muscles in the arms and shoulders. To avoid tension in the neck and upper back, always try to keep the shoulders down and relaxed.

Start with a 15 minute walk. If you are able to stay within your training zone (see page 79), gradually work your way to 30-40 minutes at least 3 times a week.

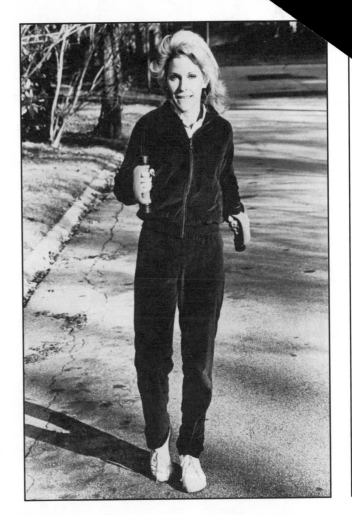

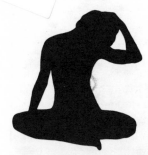

YOUR OVERALL HEALTH: PHYSICAL AND MENTAL

The Psychological Derivative
Exercise as Psychotherapy
The Biochemical Explanation

THE PSYCHOLOGICAL DERIVATIVE

You have now learned how and why to exercise for cardiovascular conditioning, strength and flexibility. Most important may be what exercise can do for your psychological outlook.

Don't be misled by my enthusiasm for exercise. If you have been sedentary since your back pain began, your body may revolt if you begin too much exercise all at once. Adhere to the conservative number of repetitions and add one new exercise a day. The first month or two will be difficult but after that, your activities will become easier, more enjoyable, and (hopefully) addictive. After my ordeal, I was so grateful to be able to sit and walk again that I cherished (and still do) the "opportunity" to exercise.

Exercise can be a way of life, a means by which you do all that you can do for "yourself," your body, and your mind. Exercise can also be therapy, not just for the musculoskeletal system, but for common anxieties, depression, low self-esteem and poor self-concept related to body image.

A person sick with the flu often may feel irritable and depressed. This is a simple example of the mind-body connection. I believe that because there is a strong relationship between psychological and physiological function, there is an equally strong relationship between psychotherapy and physical activity.

EXERCISE AS PSYCHOTHERAPY

If you choose to view exercise as therapy for your emotional well-being, begin by thinking of it as a lifestyle conversion, not a fitness program. It is a commitment you make to yourself, needing no one but yourself.

Researchers have found that as physical fitness increases, depression and anxiety decrease. An improvement in self-concept may be one explanation. Theoretically, a person's body image exerts a central influence on self-concept. It is not so much what you can do, it is how much more you can do than you did say, the month before. If you compete only with yourself and you are faithful to your program, you will be a winner every time.

Exercise fulfills many inherent needs. The need for movement, self-assertion, mastery over what we perceive as a difficult task. It helps us to play, meditate and lose ourselves in something greater than ourselves. This is particularly true of aerobic activity, where the body sustains motion over a period of time. Anxiety may be relieved because of the relaxing effect of exercise. After a workout there is a pleasant fatigue combined with a sense of accomplishment. One also sleeps better and awakes more rested after exercising during the day.

Another important psychological derivative is enhanced self-esteem. Self-esteem can be altered by anxiety and depression. If we are anxious or depressed, we do not feel good about ourselves.

Self-esteem is also determined by the ratio of success to failure. This is why it is so important that every individual have his or her own fitness program and individual goals. During daily exercise, we choose the place, the time, the pace, the goal. We regain our initiative, our sense of power. We are in control.

The mental and physical strength we develop from exercise can overpower weaknesses in other areas of our lives. Our self-produced mastery of a difficult task can be generalized, for example, to our jobs. This "strength" allows us to get in touch with our whole being — our inner selves — through our exterior selves, giving us a sense of security.

THE BIOCHEMICAL EXPLANATION

Physicians and psychologists are studying physiological evidence which indicates that aerobic exercise, done regularly for sustained periods, may stimulate the production of certain body chemicals that can have the same effects as anti-depressant drugs.

For example, certain depressions may be associated with a relative deficiency of norepinephrine at the receptor sites in the brain, while elation may be associated with an excess of this chemical. Epinephine and norepinephrine (known as adrenalin) are known to be liberated during aerobic activity and may stimulate the brain to secrete endorphins. Endorphins are naturally-occurring morphine-like substances which are found in the limbic brain region — an area known to control emotion. Long duration of aerobic activity may increase the production of endorphins, combating physical pain and fatigue and turning it to euphoria.

This euphoria or "high" has been most frequently reported from long-distance runners. However, you too can experience it on your stationary bike, in the pool, or during your walk if you work hard and long enough.

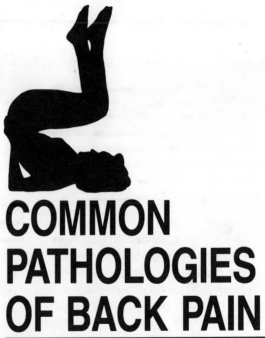

COMMON PATHOLOGIES OF BACK PAIN

Muscle Strain
Ligamentous Sprain
Nerve Root Compression
Sciatica
Biomechanical Factors
Osteoporosis

COMMON PATHOLOGIES

Low back pain occurs frequently and is chiefly a result of the manner in which this area of the body is constructed and treated or (more aptly stated), mistreated. The spine must support the weight of the body and yet be able to bend or twist in any direction. The curve of the lower back is reversed from the rest of the spine. When you stand up, weight is borne on the small joints of your back's vertebrae, instead of on the large columnar bodies in the front of the vertebrae that were designed to support the weight. Therefore, a person with swayback is more susceptible to back strain.

I have saved this material for this part of the book partly because of its complexity but primarily because the road to health must be a positive one. It is important to understand what causes pain, but it is even more important to learn how to prevent it.

Use the following information for reference. Diagnosis is the responsibility of your doctor or physical therapist. These are but a **few** of the many causes of back pain:

- Muscle strain
- Ligamentous sprain
- Sciatic nerve pain
- Biomechanical factors
- Osteoporosis

The etiology of **muscle strain** is often obscure, because there are many possible causes. Most often, a strain is caused by overuse, an abnormal muscular contraction, or strength imbalance of the muscles. Or the cause could be mineral imbalance caused by profuse sweating or diuretics and/or fatigue metabolites collected in the muscle itself. Detection of the injury is accomplished by understanding how the injury occurred and the administration of a muscle test to determine the specific locality. The following are signs that may indicate a strain:

- a "snapping" sound when the tissue tears
- complaint of muscle fatigue and spasm
- a severe loss of function or weakness of the affected part
- a spasmodic muscle contraction of the affected part
- extreme point-tenderness if touched (if surface muscle)
- a sharp pain immediately upon the occurrence of an injury

Continued stretching of a strained muscle could lead to chronic inflammation. If you experience any of these symptoms, do not attempt physical work or exercise.

Sprain by contrast, is damage to the ligaments, the connectors that bind joints. Sprains occur when ligaments are partially or completely torn, and the harm is usually done through an accident or because of a sudden blow, the kind often suffered in sports. In the back, any weakening or failure of a ligament may cause further damage by leaving the joint improperly aligned, endangering the facets, discs, or vertebrae. A sprain also generally takes longer to heal. Sometimes a strain will lead to or directly cause a sprain, as when a strained muscle is weak and unable to support the joint.

For example, someone who has a lumbosacral sprain will experience a diffused, dull ache in the lower back that is caused by an irritation of the 5th lumbar nerve. Other symptoms may be spasm, point tenderness and restricted trunk movement. In the acute stages, the pain can be incapacitating with only the slightest relief coming from lying on the floor with the knees pulled into the chest, or doing the abdominal stretch on page 55.

The initial treatment in the acute stage of severe strains or sprains is often complete bedrest, anti-inflammatory medication, ice progressing to heat, and (possibly) 90/90 traction. The individual must stay in bed until the pain no longer persists in an acute state. Return to movement, even mild activities, should be under the watchful eyes and care of a physician and physical therapist.

A pioneer orthopedic surgeon in the field of conservative treatment of low back pain, Dr. Paul C. Williams, has suggested that most athletic young persons have at least a tear in the annulus (the ligament which holds discs in place) by the time they are 20 years old. Over a period of time, if the person remains physically active, he or she will probably go on to complete the rupture of the ligament around the disc, allowing some of the rubbery, jelly-like substance between the vertebral bodies to extrude under pressure. This material may be forced out from between the vertebral bodies and impinge on the lumbar nerves. This pinching of the nerves by the disc fragment usually leads to extreme pain in the low back, buttocks, and down the back or side of the thigh into the leg and foot if the compression is severe enough. The distribution of this pain is characteristic and follows the route of the sciatic nerve, and the condition is commonly known as a "disc bulge."

Acute **nerve root compression** in the lumbar spine tends to produce a particular set of symptoms. There is usually pain and stiffness in the area of the low back where the nerve compression is taking place. This causes a muscle spasm as a protective reaction over the injured nerve root. This muscle spasm causes the person to walk bent forward at the waist, leaning to one side to avoid stretching. In severe cases the person may be unable to stand at all.

Sciatica is the pathological term used to describe the inflamed condition of the sciatic nerve which produces pain, tingling, or numbness. This nerve is vulnerable to torsions or direct blows that tend to produce abnormal stretching and pressure on it as it emerges from the spine. The sciatic nerve is also subject to trauma where it crosses over the ischial spine (base of pelvis). There, a muscle spasm or a direct blow can place pressure on the nerve.

Biomechanical factors are of the greatest importance in understanding how low back pain develops. The trouble arises from the areas of the spine subjected to the heaviest mechanical stress. Many sports subject the spine to potentially harmful stresses.

- Weight-loading sports, which tend to compress the spine, include not only weight lifting, but bowling, horseback riding, motorbiking, and jogging on hard surfaces.
- Rotatory activities subject the spine to a forceful twist. Among them are squash, racketball, tennis, batting a baseball, and golf.
- Back-arching sports include skiing, tennis, volleyball, basketball, rowing, archery, and two swimming strokes — the breast stroke and the butterfly.

There are several other lifestyle variables that, when coupled with overuse or improper training, can predispose an athlete to injury. Psychosocial factors, or stresses such as alcoholism, divorce, job dissatisfaction or an otherwise disturbed personality have been said to be responsible for 80% of low back pain. Working conditions that require repeated lifting of heavy loads, forward stooping positions and sudden stresses increase pain because they increase mechanical loads on the spine.

Osteoporosis is a condition that occurs in the latter years. The victims are most often women who have passed menopause. The vertebrae become abnormally thin and vulnerable to fracture and compression. The causes are disuse, typically in a person confined to bed for a long time without exercise or years of low physical activity, and the loss of estrogen and calcium. There is a constant turnover of calcium within bone. If an adequate amount of calcium is not supplied by the diet, calcium will be mobilized from the bones into the bloodstream.

At first there may be pain in the spine, but as the disease progresses "dowager's hump" or "widow's hump" may appear. The posture becomes more stooped and height decreases as a result of bone settling.

The best way to handle osteoporosis is to prevent it.

Your best defenses:

- Eat a low protein diet. Protein interferes with the body's ability to absorb calcium.
- Cut out soft drinks. Sodas are high in phosphoric acids, which inhibit the absorption of calcium.
- Eat a calcium-rich diet. Green leafy vegetables and dairy products are good sources.
- Estrogen supplements (for post-menopausal women with no history of cancer).
- A 1000 mg calcium carbonate supplement — with your physician's approval!
- Exercise! You actually keep your bones strong by working your muscles, because of the pull contracting muscles have on bone. Weight-bearing activities, such as walking, help maintain strong bones.

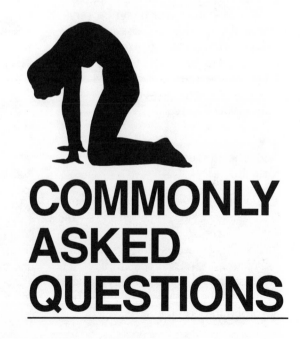

COMMONLY
ASKED
QUESTIONS

Q Why is fiber important in my diet?

A Fiber is critical to maintaining proper functioning of the digestive system and elimination. By adding fiber to the diet (such as bran flakes), you decrease the transit time of your food. This helps prevent constipation, which can be very painful if you have disc disease.

Be sure to eat the skin on apples and potatoes, eat plenty of steamed vegetables, whole grain bread, pastas and rice. Add 1 tablespoon of bran flakes to your morning cereal.

Q When do I use heat on an injury or for pain?

A Do not use heat on a sprain for the first 72 hours, or inflammation and swelling will increase. Wet heat is excellent for sore, tight muscles, strained muscles, old injuries, and muscle spasms. Dry heating pads may relax you but they are not as therapeutic. Only wet heat can be absorbed through the skin.

Q What kind of shoes should I wear to walk long distances?

A Provide your spine with as much protection as possible when you walk. Look for shoes with:
- Maximal shock absorption (thick soles with deep tread).
- Plenty of lateral support (lateral leather uppers).
- Sturdy heel counters (back of heel support).

Take this description to an athletic shoe store and have an expert fit you with good, sturdy shoes. Tell the salesperson you'll use the shoes for walking.

Q When do I use ice for an injury or for pain?

A Ice is recommended for the first 72 hours if you have a sprain or pulled muscle. The ice pack should not be left on one spot for longer than 20 minutes at a time. Ice is an excellent analgesic and anti-inflammatory, and also can be used effectively on a muscle spasm.

Q Sexual intercourse hurts my back. What is the safest position for me?

A A back pain sufferer must lie on one side or assume the dominant position, because hip adduction plus the weight of your partner places enormous stress upon the ligaments of the pelvis.

Q When should I wear a lumbar support brace?

A As seldom as possible, and only on the advice of your orthopedist. A brace is a wonderful support when you have to stand or sit for long periods or when performing household chores such as vacuuming. If abused or overused, a brace will leave your back muscles very weak. This is because when you wear the brace it takes the place of your muscles in supporting your body. It is true: if you don't use them you will lose them. This axiom is most applicable to muscle strength.

Hot Soak in tub

Q **What is the safest way to lose weight?**

A Gradually, combining your exercise with a 500-calorie decrease in your daily calorie intake. No matter what you've heard, calories do count. In order to keep up with them, use a calorie reference book and write them down as you consume them.

Cut out white flour and sugar. Foods made from these substances have very little nutritional value and are high in calories. Eat complex carbohydrates.

Cut down on saturated fats and eat only dairy products that are marked lowfat.

Don't skip meals. This only leads to a fall in blood sugar which makes you hungrier for high sugar foods. The best meal plan to stimulate digestion and metabolism is six small feedings a day of approximately 200 calories each, eaten every 3 hours.

Drink 8 glasses of water a day. Water will flush toxins from your body and leave you with a "full" feeling.

Q **What carbohydrate foods are "complex?"**

A These are foods such as legumes, grains, fruits, and vegetables. Once these carbohydrate foods are digested, they are transformed into glucose which supplies the body with a long lasting supply of energy. Even if you are on a diet, at least 60% of your calories should come from complex carbohydrates. It is not the potato (90 calories) or the piece of whole wheat bread (80 calories) that are so "fattening." It is the one tablespoon of butter (100 calories from fat) that you put on them that add up. We all need carbohydrates for energy!

Q **What are proteins?**

A They are the building blocks of the cells in every body tissue. However, your diet need contain only 20% protein. This can be obtained from lowfat dairy products, tofu, eggs, chicken, fish and combinations of legumes and whole grains. You don't need red meat every day. Beef is high in saturated fat, which has been linked to heart disease. Think about getting your protein from lowfat cottage cheese in the morning, plain lowfat yogurt with fruit for lunch, and baked fish for dinner. Now that is low fat and low calories!

Q **So why is fat so bad?**

A Fats contain 9 calories per gram, carbohydrates and proteins contain 4 calories per gram. It's easy to see how a diet high in fat could cause you to put on pounds. A high fat diet has also been linked to high blood pressure, heart and artery disease, colon and breast cancer, and excessive weight gain. Some fat is necessary. One tablespoon of safflower or sunflower oil daily will fill your requirement for essential fatty acids.

Q Will my muscles get sore and, if so, why?

A An inevitable result of resuming exercise after a period of inactivity is muscle soreness. Acute soreness is thought to be associated with inadequate blood flow (ischemia) caused by a forceful muscle contraction. The resulting sensation is burning and cramping, caused by a buildup of lactic acid. Lactic acid is removed from the muscle within 30 minutes and pain then dissipates, but delayed soreness doesn't occur until 24-36 hours have passed. The most accepted theory by physiologists of delayed muscle soreness is the tissue damage theory. Evidence shows that intense exercise damages muscle fibers and surrounding connective tissue. These tissues become swollen and painful. The pain causes a reflex muscle spasm which constricts blood vessels and shunts blood flow.

Q What are effective remedies for muscle spasm?

A The most effective remedies are wet heat and massage. Therapeutic sports massage is the practice of deep, direct-applied pressure, friction and compression to spread constricted fibers. This enlarges capillaries, enhancing blood flow to the affected area. The increased blood supply acts as a natural analgesic. The type of stroke applied and the amount of pressure used is determined by the severity of the soreness and whether or not discomfort is being caused by a muscle spasm in a specific area.

Have a friend palpate deeply on your back until the most tender spot is located. If it is not on a bone, have the friend apply sustained pressure into this tender spot until the muscle releases. The pressure will be uncomfortable but should not be so intense that it elicits pain. The direct pressure will inhibit the nerve response to the spinal cord that is signaling the muscle to spasm. This could take anywhere from 2 minutes to 1 hour. More treatment may be needed.

Direct pressure may be alternated with kneading of the adjacent muscles (similar to the way one works with bread dough). If you would like to have professional massage, look in the Yellow Pages under Massage Therapy. Look for a licensed M.T., massage therapist, from an accredited school. Check to see if the therapist has been trained in sports massage.

Caution: Don't let a massage therapist manipulate your joints. Tell him or her ahead of time you don't want manipulation. Most massage therapists are not trained to do this and may do you more harm than good.

Q How often should I exercise?

A In the beginning, I recommend that you alternate your aerobic days with your calisthenic days. Walk Monday, Wednesday, Friday; do calisthenics on Tuesday, Thursday, and Saturday. Take Sunday off. As you get stronger, try doing both workouts five days a week. It is always advisable for even the healthiest athlete to take at least one day off a week and rest!

Q What about wearing high-heeled shoes?

A Don't, even when walking short distances. Heels higher than 1½ inches shift your body weight forward and exaggerate your lordosis.

Q What is the best way to lift a heavy suitcase?

A There is not a safe way. Try a suitcase with rollers or have someone help you.

Q It hurts when I cough or sneeze. Is there anything I can do?

A Yes, stand up, hold your stomach muscles in as tightly as possible and lean slightly backward. Bend your knees.

Q I not only have pain in my back but in my elbow and shoulder too. Could they be related?

A Yes. All undiagnosed joint pain should be evaluated by a rheumatologist. Arthritic conditions can and should be treated.

Q Can a psychologist help me deal with my pain?

A Most definitely! Stress management is very important in preventing and dealing with back pain. If you are unable to seek professional help for financial reasons, a very effective alternative can be a stress management cassette tape. Listening to the tape every morning and evening or when you are in pain can help muscles relax, help you to sleep and, most importantly, help you approach each day with a calm sense of well being. Cassette tapes can be purchased at most bookstores.

Q I awaken during the night and feel tired all day. What can I do?

A A lot of research has been done lately on the correlation of irregular sleep patterns and muscle pain. If the normal sleep cycle is not resumed, a muscular condition called fibrositis could result. Rheumatologists commonly treat fibrositis. Therapy may be a small dose of anti-depressant medication before bedtime that will allow one to sleep through the night. If sleep is a problem for you, ask your doctor for help. If you don't get enough "restful" sleep, your muscles won't be able to rest either.

Q What's the best prescription for back pain?

A Have your doctor refer you to an orthopedic physical therapist. Hands on therapy, proper daily body mechanics, and (of course) a consistent exercise program are the best avenues you can take to a pain-free back.

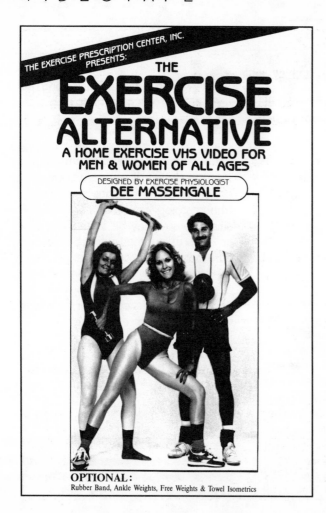

94

WHO CAN USE
THE EXERCISE ALTERNATIVE?

Everybody — from Beginners to Advanced Exercisers — can derive a satisfying workout, because the degree of difficulty depends on the amount of hand and ankle weights, if any, the user chooses. The tape is designed to develop muscle tone and strength in every major muscle group, and is 55 minutes long.

Yes! Please send me "The Exercise Alternative" on VHS.

I have enclosed a check or money order for $31.95 ($29.95 plus $2 shipping and handling) made payable to The Exercise Prescription Center, Inc.

Mail to:

The Exercise Prescription Center, Inc.
477 Bryn Mawr Lane, N.W.
Atlanta, Ga. 30327

Name_____

Address_____

_____

City_____

State_____ Zip_____

WHY IS IT CALLED THE EXERCISE ALTERNATIVE? WHAT MAKES IT DIFFERENT?

It is called the exercise alternative because there are no running, jumping, or joint compression exercises, and because each exercise is thoroughly explained. Dee shows you how to stretch before a muscle fatigues, and gives alternatives for difficult exercises. Her #1 priority is safety and preventing joint-related stress and injuries.

95